Acupressure Healing Guide for Beginners

Incorporating Acupressure into Daily Living

By

Delaney Erick

Copyright@2023

Table of Contents

CHAPTER 1
Introduction

Acupressure is an ancient healing practice that has its roots in traditional Chinese medicine (TCM). It is a holistic approach to health and wellness that involves the application of manual pressure to specific points on the body to stimulate the body's natural healing abilities. This therapeutic technique has been used for thousands of years and is based on the belief that the body's vital energy, known as "Qi" (pronounced "chee"), flows through a network of channels or meridians. Acupressure seeks to balance and harmonize the flow of Qi to promote physical, emotional, and mental well-being.

1.1 What is Acupressure?

Acupressure is often described as acupuncture without needles. Instead of using needles, acupressure relies on the application of firm yet gentle pressure to specific acupoints on the body's surface. These acupoints are located along the meridians or energy pathways and are believed to correspond to various organs, systems, and functions of the body. By stimulating these points, acupressure aims to restore balance and alleviate a wide range of health issues, from pain and discomfort to emotional stress and fatigue.

Acupressure techniques can vary, but they typically involve using fingers, thumbs, or specialized tools to exert pressure on the acupoints. The amount of pressure, duration, and frequency of the treatment can be adjusted to suit individual needs and preferences. Acupressure is non-invasive, safe, and can be easily learned and applied by individuals for self-care or administered by trained practitioners.

1.2 How Does Acupressure Work?

The fundamental principle behind acupressure is the concept of Qi and the meridian system. According to TCM, Qi is the vital life force that flows through the body, nourishing and supporting all its functions. When Qi becomes blocked or imbalanced, it can result in various physical or emotional ailments. Acupressure works by promoting the free flow of Qi and restoring balance along the meridians.

By applying pressure to specific acupoints, acupressure can:

- **Relieve Tension and Pain:** Acupressure is particularly effective in alleviating muscle tension and pain. It can be used to address issues such as headaches, neck and back pain, and menstrual cramps.

- **Reduce Stress and Anxiety:** The calming effect of acupressure can help reduce stress and anxiety by triggering the release of endorphins, the body's natural painkillers, and promoting relaxation.

- **Enhance Circulation:** Acupressure can improve blood circulation, which is essential for overall health and healing.

Improved circulation can help with
issues like cold hands and feet.

- **Boost Immunity:** By stimulating
  specific acupoints, acupressure can
  enhance the body's natural defense
  mechanisms, making it more
  resilient to illnesses.

- **Balance Emotions:** Acupressure
  is not just about physical healing;
  it can also address emotional
  imbalances. It can help regulate
  mood, improve sleep, and promote
  a sense of well-being.

- **Support Digestion:** Acupressure
  can aid in digestive health by
  relieving symptoms of indigestion,
  bloating, and constipation.

1.3 Benefits of Acupressure

Acupressure offers a wide range of benefits that extend beyond physical health. Some of the key benefits include:

- **Natural Healing:** Acupressure is a non-invasive and drug-free approach to healing, making it suitable for individuals seeking natural remedies.

- **Holistic Wellness:** It addresses the mind-body connection, recognizing that emotional and mental well-being are interconnected with physical health.

- **Complementary Therapy:** Acupressure can complement other forms of treatment, including

conventional medicine, physical
therapy, and counseling, enhancing
overall care.

- **Self-Care:** Many acupressure
  techniques are simple enough for
  individuals to learn and practice on
  themselves, empowering them to
  take control of their health and
  well-being.

- **Cost-Effective:** Acupressure is a
  cost-effective therapy that doesn't
  require expensive equipment or
  ongoing expenses.

acupressure is a time-tested healing
modality that offers a holistic
approach to health and well-being. It
works by balancing the body's energy
flow, promoting relaxation, and
supporting natural healing processes.
With its numerous benefits, it has
gained popularity worldwide as a

complementary and alternative therapy for a wide range of health concerns. Whether you're a beginner or an experienced practitioner, acupressure can be a valuable tool in your journey toward improved health and vitality.

1.4 Safety Precautions

While acupressure is generally considered safe, it's essential to follow some safety precautions to ensure a positive and risk-free experience. Here are some key safety guidelines to keep in mind when practicing acupressure:

1. **Consult a Healthcare Professional:** If you have any underlying medical conditions, are pregnant, or are taking medications, consult with a

qualified healthcare professional before starting acupressure. They can provide guidance on whether acupressure is suitable for your specific situation.

2. **Learn Proper Techniques:** It's crucial to learn and understand the correct acupressure techniques. Incorrect application of pressure or targeting the wrong acupoints can lead to discomfort or adverse effects.

3. **Start Gently:** If you're new to acupressure, begin with gentle pressure and gradually increase it as you become more comfortable with the practice. Avoid using excessive force, as it may cause bruising or discomfort.

4. **Pain vs. Discomfort:** Pay attention to your body's response.

Acupressure should not be painful. You may experience some mild discomfort, but if you feel sharp pain or severe discomfort, stop immediately and reevaluate your technique.

5. **Avoid Open Wounds or Skin Conditions:** Do not apply acupressure to areas with open wounds, cuts, rashes, or skin conditions. It's essential to work on clean and healthy skin to prevent infection or irritation.

6. **Avoid Certain Points During Pregnancy:** Some acupressure points are contraindicated during pregnancy, as they may stimulate uterine contractions. Pregnant individuals should seek guidance from a healthcare provider or a qualified acupressure practitioner.

7. **Hygiene and Cleanliness:** Ensure that your hands and the area you're working on are clean and hygienic to prevent infection.

8. **Use the Right Tools:** If you're using acupressure tools, such as rollers or balls, ensure they are of high quality and safe for use on the skin. Clean and sanitize your tools regularly.

9. **Stay Hydrated:** After an acupressure session, it's a good practice to drink water to help flush out any toxins released during the treatment.

10. **Monitor for Side Effects:** Pay attention to any adverse reactions, such as dizziness, nausea, or increased pain, during or after an acupressure session. If you experience any concerning

symptoms, discontinue the practice and seek medical advice if needed.

11. **Individual Variations:** Every individual is unique, and what works for one person may not work for another. Pay attention to how your body responds to acupressure and adjust your practice accordingly.

12. **Seek Professional Guidance:** If you have a specific health condition or ailment you want to address with acupressure, consider consulting with a qualified acupressure practitioner who can provide personalized guidance and treatment plans.

Acupressure is a complementary therapy and should not be used as a sole substitute for medical treatment when necessary. Safety and self-awareness are paramount in acupressure practice, and it's essential to prioritize your well-being throughout your acupressure journey.

CHAPTER 2

Understanding the Basics

Acupressure is an ancient healing art that relies on the manipulation of specific points on the body to promote health and alleviate various conditions. To grasp the fundamentals of acupressure, it's essential to understand acupressure points and meridians, the tools and equipment used, and the importance of proper body posture during practice.

2.1 Acupressure Points and Meridians

Acupressure Points: Acupressure points, also known as acupoints, are specific locations on the body's surface where acupressure techniques are applied. These points are typically found along pathways known as meridians or channels. Acupoints are the focal points for directing energy (Qi) flow in the body. There are hundreds of acupoints throughout the body, each with its unique properties and functions.

Meridians: Meridians are energy pathways that run through the body, similar to the circulatory system but carrying Qi, the vital life force, instead of blood. There are twelve primary meridians, each associated with a specific organ or body system. These meridians provide the blueprint for understanding how Qi flows through the body. Acupressure aims to balance and harmonize the flow of Qi in these meridians to promote health and well-being.

2.2 Tools and Equipment

Fingers and Thumbs: The most commonly used tools in acupressure are your own fingers and thumbs. They provide precise control over pressure application and are readily available for self-treatment. Fingers and thumbs are used to apply pressure to acupoints to stimulate or calm energy flow.

Acupressure Tools: Some individuals prefer to use specialized tools designed for acupressure, such as acupressure balls, rollers, or mats. These tools can help distribute pressure evenly and may be especially useful for specific conditions or hard-to-reach areas. When using acupressure tools, it's essential to follow the manufacturer's instructions and apply gentle pressure.

2.3 Proper Body Posture

Sitting or Lying Down: Proper body posture is essential during acupressure practice to ensure comfort and effectiveness. When performing acupressure on yourself or others, sit or lie down in a relaxed position. A comfortable chair, yoga mat, or massage table can be used as a surface for acupressure.

Alignment: Maintain good body alignment by keeping your spine straight and shoulders relaxed. This helps prevent unnecessary strain on your back and neck.

Relaxed Muscles: Tension in your body can interfere with the flow of Qi. Therefore, it's essential to keep your muscles relaxed while applying pressure to acupoints. Breathe deeply and slowly to encourage relaxation.

Focus on the Point: When applying pressure to an acupoint, focus your intention and attention on that specific point. Concentrate on your breathing and visualize the energy flowing through the meridian.

Comfort and Support: Use cushions or props to support your body and make the acupressure process more comfortable, especially during longer sessions.

Understanding the basics of acupressure, including acupoints, meridians, tools, and proper body posture, forms the foundation for safe and effective practice. These fundamentals empower individuals to explore acupressure for self-care and well-being, helping them harness the potential benefits of this ancient healing art.

CHAPTER 3

Getting Started with Acupressure

Before you begin your journey into acupressure, it's important to prepare yourself mentally and physically for the practice. Here we will cover the essential steps for starting acupressure, including preparing yourself, mastering breathing and relaxation techniques, and setting intentions.

3.1 Preparing Yourself

Preparing yourself is a crucial step to ensure a successful and enjoyable acupressure experience. Here's how you can prepare:

- **Choose a Quiet Space:** Find a quiet and comfortable space where you can practice acupressure without disturbances. This will help you focus and relax.

- **Gather Supplies:** If you're using any specific tools or equipment for acupressure, make sure they're readily available and within reach.

- **Dress Comfortably:** Wear loose, comfortable clothing that allows for easy movement. This will help you maintain proper body posture during the practice.

- **Empty Stomach:** It's generally best to practice acupressure on an empty stomach or a few hours after a meal to avoid discomfort or nausea.

- **Silence Your Devices:** Turn off or silence your phone and other electronic devices to minimize distractions.

- **Set Aside Time:** Allocate enough time for your acupressure session. Rushing through the practice can be counterproductive. Start with a manageable duration, and as you become more experienced, you can extend your sessions.

3.2 Breathing and Relaxation Techniques

Proper breathing and relaxation are integral to acupressure practice. These techniques help you calm your mind, reduce stress, and enhance the effectiveness of the treatment:

- **Deep Breathing:** Begin your acupressure session with a few minutes of deep, slow breathing. Inhale deeply through your nose, allowing your abdomen to expand, and exhale slowly through your mouth. Focus on your breath and let go of any tension with each exhale.

- **Progressive Muscle Relaxation:** Before applying pressure to acupoints, take a moment to mentally scan your body. Start from your toes and work your way up, consciously relaxing each muscle group. This helps create a state of relaxation.

- **Mindfulness Meditation:** Incorporating mindfulness meditation techniques can be beneficial. Pay close attention to the sensations in your body as you apply pressure to acupoints. This mindfulness can enhance your awareness of the body's responses.

3.3 Setting Intentions

Setting intentions is a powerful aspect of acupressure practice. It helps you focus your mind and energy on specific goals or outcomes:

- **Clarify Your Goals:** Before beginning, take a moment to clarify your intentions for the acupressure session. Are you seeking pain relief, stress reduction, improved sleep, or emotional balance? Understanding your goals will guide your practice.

- **Visualize the Outcome:** Close your eyes and visualize the desired outcome of your acupressure session. Imagine yourself feeling relaxed, pain-free, or emotionally balanced. This visualization can help manifest your intentions.

- **Affirmations:** Consider using positive affirmations related to your intentions. Repeat these affirmations silently or aloud during the session to reinforce your goals.

- **Stay Open to the Experience:** While it's important to have clear intentions, also remain open to the unexpected benefits of acupressure. Sometimes, the practice may provide solutions or insights beyond your initial goals.

Preparing yourself, mastering breathing and relaxation techniques, and setting clear intentions, you can enhance the effectiveness of your acupressure practice. These steps create a conducive environment for healing and self-care, allowing you to experience the full benefits of this ancient therapeutic art.

CHAPTER 4

Common Acupressure Points

Acupressure involves stimulating specific points on the body to promote healing and alleviate various symptoms. Here we'll explore common acupressure points grouped by different regions of the body.

4.1 Head and Neck Points

Acupressure points in the head and neck region are often used to relieve tension, headaches, and stress:

Third Eye Point (GV24.5): Located between the eyebrows, in the indentation just above the bridge of the nose. Stimulating this point can help relieve headaches, improve concentration, and reduce stress.

Heavenly Pillar (B10): Situated on the back of the neck, one thumb-width below the base of the skull on either side of the spine. Massaging these points can alleviate neck pain, tension, and headaches.

Drilling Bamboo (B2): Found in the hollows on either side of the bridge of the nose, near the inner corners of the eyebrows. Gently applying pressure to these points can help relieve sinus congestion and eye strain.

Wind Pool (GB20): Located in the hollows on both sides of the neck, where the neck muscles attach to the base of the skull. Stimulating these points can relieve headaches, neck pain, and stress.

4.2 Upper Body Points

These acupressure points are situated in the upper body and can be useful for conditions like shoulder pain, anxiety, and respiratory issues:

Shoulder Well (GB21): Found on the tops of the shoulders, midway between the base of the neck and the outer edge of the shoulders. Massaging this point can help relieve shoulder and neck tension.

Sea of Tranquility (CV17): Located in the center of the breastbone, at the level of the fourth rib. Pressing this point can help reduce anxiety, stress, and chest congestion.

Lung 1 (LU1): Situated on the upper chest, three finger-widths below the collarbone. Stimulating this point can ease respiratory issues, coughing, and chest tightness.

4.3 Lower Body Points

These acupressure points in the lower body are beneficial for addressing issues like lower back pain, digestion, and menstrual discomfort:

Lower Sea of Energy (CV6): Located two finger-widths below the navel. Applying pressure to this point can improve digestion, relieve menstrual pain, and boost overall energy.

Sacral Points (B48): Found on either side of the spine, just above the sacrum (the triangular bone at the base of the spine). Massaging these points can help alleviate lower back pain and sciatica.

Leg Three Miles (ST36): Situated about four finger-widths below the kneecap and one finger-width towards the outside of the shinbone. Stimulating this point can boost energy, aid digestion, and relieve knee pain.

4.4 Hand and Foot Points

Acupressure points in the hands and feet are accessible and useful for various conditions:

Great Rushing (LV3): Located on the top of the foot, in the hollow between the big toe and the second toe. Massaging this point can help alleviate stress, reduce anger, and improve the flow of Qi.

Joining Valley (LI4): Found in the webbing between the thumb and index finger on both hands. Stimulating this point can relieve headaches, sinus congestion, and promote relaxation.

Bigger Stream (K3): Situated on the inner side of the foot, in the hollow between the ankle bone and the Achilles tendon. Pressing this point can help with insomnia, anxiety, and lower back pain.

These are just a few common acupressure points across different regions of the body. When using acupressure, it's essential to apply gentle yet firm pressure and hold each point for 1 to 3 minutes while focusing on your breath and relaxation. It's also advisable to consult with a qualified acupressure practitioner or healthcare provider for personalized guidance and to ensure that acupressure is appropriate for your specific needs.

CHAPTER 5

Techniques and Methods

Acupressure involves various techniques and methods for applying pressure to specific points on the body.

5.1 Finger and Thumb Pressure

Finger and thumb pressure is the most common and basic acupressure technique. It involves using your fingers, thumbs, or both to apply controlled pressure to acupoints. Here's a step-by-step guide on how to perform finger and thumb pressure acupressure:

Preparation:

1. **Choose a Comfortable Position:** Sit or lie down in a comfortable and relaxed position. Ensure that the area you want to treat is easily accessible.

2. **Relaxation:** Take a few deep breaths to relax your body and calm your mind. This will enhance the effectiveness of the acupressure.

3. **Locate the Acupoint:** Use a reference guide or chart to locate the specific acupoint you want to work on. Acupoints are typically identified by their names and coordinates.

Application of Finger and Thumb Pressure:

4. **Use Your Fingers or Thumbs:**
   Depending on the location and size
   of the acupoint, you can use either
   your fingers or thumbs to apply
   pressure. Use the part of your
   finger or thumb that's most
   comfortable and feels most
   effective for the specific point.

5. **Apply Firm Yet Gentle
   Pressure:** Position your finger or
   thumb directly on the acupoint and
   apply firm, steady pressure. The
   pressure should be enough to feel a
   slight discomfort or "good pain,"
   but it should not be painful. The
   sensation should be tolerable and
   should not cause bruising or
   injury.

6. **Circular Motion:** Once you've applied pressure, you can use a circular motion with your finger or thumb to stimulate the acupoint. Move in a clockwise direction while maintaining the pressure. This circular motion helps activate the energy flow in the meridian.

7. **Duration:** Hold the pressure on the acupoint for 1 to 3 minutes. During this time, focus on your breath and try to relax. As you hold the pressure, you may feel a sense of warmth, tingling, or relaxation in the area.

8. **Release Slowly:** After the recommended time, release the pressure slowly and gently. You can repeat this process several times, gradually increasing the pressure if needed.

9. **Rest:** Give yourself a few moments to rest and observe any changes in the area. It's common to feel relief, relaxation, or improved energy flow after an acupressure session.

Tips:

- Always start with gentle pressure and gradually increase it if necessary. Avoid using excessive force to prevent discomfort or injury.

- Use a comfortable body posture to maintain proper alignment and reduce strain during the practice.

- If you're working on multiple acupoints, focus on one at a time to ensure that you're giving each point adequate attention.

- Be patient and consistent with your acupressure practice. It may take time to see significant results, especially for chronic conditions.

- Consult a qualified acupressure practitioner or reference guide to identify the most effective acupoints for your specific needs.

Finger and thumb pressure is a versatile acupressure technique that you can use for self-care and to address a wide range of physical and emotional concerns. It's a safe and accessible method that, when performed correctly, can provide relief and promote overall well-being.

5.2 Circular Motion

Circular motion is a technique commonly used in acupressure to stimulate acupoints and meridians. This method involves applying pressure with your fingers or thumbs in a circular, rotating motion over a specific acupoint. Here's a detailed explanation of how to use circular motion in acupressure:

Preparation:

1. **Choose the Acupoint:** First, identify the acupoint you want to work on using a reference guide or chart. Note its location and any specific conditions it can address.

Application of Circular Motion:

2. **Position Your Finger or Thumb:** Place your finger or

thumb directly on the acupoint. Ensure your hand is relaxed, and your fingers are comfortably positioned to allow for circular motion.

3. **Apply Steady Pressure:** Begin by applying steady but gentle pressure to the acupoint. The pressure should be firm enough to feel some discomfort or a sensation often described as "good pain." However, it should not be painful, and it should not cause bruising.

4. **Start the Circular Motion:** While maintaining pressure, start moving your finger or thumb in a circular motion. The circles should be small and focused on the acupoint itself. Move in a clockwise direction

to follow the natural flow of energy in the meridian.

5. **Maintain Rhythm and Pace:** Keep the circular motion steady, rhythmic, and at a comfortable pace. You can adjust the speed and size of the circles to suit your comfort and the sensitivity of the acupoint.

6. **Duration:** Continue the circular motion for about 1 to 3 minutes. During this time, focus on your breath and try to relax. Pay attention to any sensations in the area, such as warmth, tingling, or a sense of relaxation.

7. **Release Slowly:** After the recommended time, release the pressure and stop the circular motion slowly and gently. Take

a moment to rest and observe
any changes in the acupoint or
your overall well-being.

Tips:

- Start with gentle pressure and
  gradually increase it if needed.
  The key is to apply enough
  pressure to stimulate the
  acupoint effectively without
  causing discomfort or harm.

- If you're working on multiple
  acupoints, focus on one at a
  time to ensure proper attention
  and effectiveness.

- Circular motion is particularly
  useful for acupoints located in
  areas where a rotating motion is
  practical, such as the arms,
  legs, and certain points on the
  torso.

- Be patient and consistent with your acupressure practice. Results may take time, especially for chronic conditions.

5.3 Using Acupressure Tools

In addition to using your fingers and thumbs, you can enhance your acupressure practice by incorporating specialized acupressure tools. These tools are designed to target acupoints more effectively and may provide a different sensory experience. Here's how to use acupressure tools:

Preparation:

1. **Select the Appropriate Tool:** Depending on your needs and preferences, choose an

acupressure tool such as an acupressure ball, roller, mat, or wand. These tools come in various shapes and sizes, so select one that suits your purpose.

2. **Identify the Acupoint:** Determine the specific acupoint you want to target with the acupressure tool. Refer to a reference guide or chart for guidance.

Application of Acupressure Tools:

3. **Position the Tool:** Place the selected acupressure tool directly on the acupoint. Ensure that it's aligned with the point you want to stimulate.

4. **Apply Pressure:** Apply gentle and controlled pressure using the tool. The amount of

pressure should be comfortable and not overly intense. You can adjust the pressure by varying the force you exert on the tool.

5. **Move or Rotate the Tool:** Depending on the type of tool, you can move it in a circular or back-and-forth motion over the acupoint. Some tools, like rollers, can be rolled along the skin to provide a massaging effect.

6. **Duration:** Continue using the acupressure tool for 1 to 3 minutes on each acupoint. Be mindful of any sensations and adjust the pressure or technique as needed.

7. **Release Slowly:** After the recommended time, release the pressure and remove the tool

slowly and gently. Take a moment to rest and observe any changes in the acupoint or your overall well-being.

Tips:

- Choose acupressure tools made of safe, hygienic materials. Clean and maintain your tools according to the manufacturer's instructions.

- Experiment with different acupressure tools to find the ones that work best for you and your specific needs.

- Incorporate acupressure tools into your regular acupressure practice for variety and enhanced effectiveness.

- If you have any concerns or specific health conditions,

consult a qualified acupressure
practitioner or healthcare
provider for guidance on using
acupressure tools safely and
effectively.

Using circular motion and
acupressure tools can enhance your
acupressure practice, making it more
versatile and effective in addressing a
wide range of physical and emotional
concerns. Remember to prioritize
comfort and safety while exploring
these techniques.

5.4 Acupressure Massage

Acupressure massage is a therapeutic
technique that combines the principles
of acupressure with massage
movements. It involves applying
pressure to specific acupoints on the
body while incorporating various

massage techniques to promote relaxation, relieve tension, and stimulate energy flow. Here's a detailed guide on how to perform acupressure massage:

Preparation:

1. **Choose a Comfortable Environment:** Find a quiet, comfortable, and well-lit space for the massage. Ensure that the room is at a comfortable temperature.

2. **Prepare the Recipient:** If you are giving someone else an acupressure massage, make sure they are comfortable and relaxed. Ask them to lie down on a massage table, bed, or comfortable surface. Provide a soft blanket or towel for covering.

Application of Acupressure Massage:

3. **Identify the Acupoints:**
Determine the specific acupoints
you want to target during the
massage. Refer to a reference
guide or chart to locate these
points.

4. **Position Yourself:** If you are the
one performing the massage, stand
or sit comfortably beside the
recipient. If you are receiving the
massage, lie down in a relaxed
position.

5. **Apply Pressure to Acupoints:**
Use your fingers, thumbs, palms,
or knuckles to apply gentle but
firm pressure to the selected
acupoints. Begin with light
pressure and gradually increase it
as needed. Ensure that the
recipient communicates their
comfort level, and adjust the
pressure accordingly.

6. **Incorporate Massage Techniques:**

- **Kneading:** Using your fingers and palms, knead the area around the acupoint in a circular motion. This technique helps relieve muscle tension and increase blood circulation.

- **Rubbing:** Use your fingers or palms to rub the area around the acupoint in a back-and-forth or circular motion. Rubbing helps warm up the muscles and enhances relaxation.

- **Tapping or Percussion:** Lightly tap or drum your fingertips or palms over the acupoint and surrounding area. This technique promotes energy flow and stimulates the nervous system.

- **Press and Release:** Apply steady pressure to the acupoint for a few seconds and then release. Repeat this press-and-release motion several times to activate the point.

- **Stretching:** Gently stretch the limbs or muscles connected to the acupoint to further release tension.

7. **Maintain a Flowing Sequence:** Create a flowing sequence by moving from one acupoint to another. Follow the natural pathways of the meridians to harmonize the energy flow in the body.

8. **Duration:** Spend 1 to 3 minutes on each acupoint, combining pressure and massage techniques.

Allow the recipient to relax and breathe deeply during the massage.

9. **Communication:** Maintain open communication with the recipient. Ask them about the pressure and any discomfort they may feel. Adjust your techniques based on their feedback.

10. **Complete the Massage:** Finish the massage by gradually reducing the pressure and performing light strokes or effleurage over the entire body to promote relaxation.

Post-Massage:

11. **Rest:** Allow the recipient to rest for a few minutes after the massage. Provide water to help flush out toxins released during the treatment.

12. **Feedback:** Encourage the recipient to share their experience and any changes in their well-being. This feedback can guide future sessions.

Acupressure massage combines the benefits of acupressure and massage therapy, making it a versatile and effective approach for relieving physical and emotional tension, improving circulation, and enhancing overall well-being. Whether you are giving or receiving an acupressure massage, it's important to prioritize comfort, communication, and relaxation throughout the session.

CHAPTER 6

Conditions and Ailments

Acupressure can be used to address a wide range of conditions and ailments by stimulating specific acupoints to promote healing and relief. In this section, we'll explore how acupressure can be applied to two common conditions:

6.1 Stress and Anxiety

Stress and anxiety are prevalent concerns in today's fast-paced world. Acupressure can offer a natural and effective way to alleviate stress and anxiety symptoms. Here's how to use acupressure for stress and anxiety relief:

- **Third Eye Point (GV24.5):**
  Located between the eyebrows,
  apply gentle pressure to this
  point using your thumb or
  forefinger. This can help relieve
  stress, calm the mind, and
  improve focus.

- **Heavenly Pillar (B10):**
  Situated on the back of the
  neck, apply firm but gentle
  pressure to both sides of this
  point, just below the base of the
  skull. This can help alleviate
  tension, stress, and headaches.

- **Great Rushing (LV3):** Found
  on the top of the foot, in the
  hollow between the big toe and
  the second toe. Apply pressure
  to this point with your thumb to
  relieve stress, promote
  relaxation, and reduce anger.

- **Inner Gate (P6):** Located on the inner forearm, about two and a half finger-widths above the wrist crease. Gently massage or apply pressure to this point to reduce anxiety, nausea, and stress.

- **Breathing Techniques:** Combine acupressure with deep, slow breathing. Inhale deeply through your nose, and exhale slowly through your mouth while focusing on the acupoints you are stimulating. This enhances relaxation.

6.2 Headaches and Migraines

Acupressure can be an effective way to relieve tension headaches and migraines without the use of medication. Here are some acupressure points for headaches and migraines:

- **Third Eye Point (GV24.5):** As mentioned earlier, apply gentle pressure to the point between the eyebrows. This can help relieve headaches and promote relaxation.

- **Wind Pool (GB20):** Found in the hollows on both sides of the neck, at the base of the skull. Apply firm pressure to these points to alleviate tension headaches and migraines.

- **Drilling Bamboo (B2):** Located in the hollows on either side of the bridge of the nose, near the inner corners of the eyebrows. Gently press these points to relieve sinus congestion and sinus headaches.

- **Union Valley (LI4):** Situated in the webbing between the thumb and index finger on both hands. Apply pressure to these points to relieve headache pain and tension.

- **Heavenly Pillar (B10):** As mentioned earlier, this point on the back of the neck can also help with headache relief.

When using acupressure for stress, anxiety, headaches, or migraines, it's important to maintain proper body posture, use gentle yet firm pressure, and focus on relaxation. Acupressure can be a valuable part of a holistic approach to managing these conditions, and consistent practice may lead to long-term relief and improved well-being. If you have chronic or severe symptoms, it's advisable to consult a healthcare professional for a comprehensive evaluation and treatment plan.

6.3 Back Pain

Acupressure can be used to alleviate back pain, whether it's due to muscle tension, stress, or other causes. Here are some acupressure points and techniques for back pain relief:

- **Lower Back Points (B23 and B47):** These points are located on the lower back, on both sides of the spine. Apply firm, circular pressure to these points to help relieve lower back pain and tension.

- **Gate of Vitality (B23):**
  Located in the lower back,
  between the second and third
  lumbar vertebrae. Applying
  pressure to this point can help
  with lower back pain and
  fatigue.

- **Sea of Energy (CV6):** Found
  below the navel, this point can
  be effective for general back
  pain relief. Apply firm pressure
  to this point to promote energy
  flow and relieve discomfort.

- **Upper Back and Shoulder
  Points:** These include points
  like Heavenly Pillar (B10) and
  Shoulder Well (GB21), as
  mentioned earlier. Massaging
  and applying pressure to these
  points can help relieve tension
  in the upper back and

shoulders, which often contributes to back pain.

6.4 Insomnia

Acupressure can be a helpful complementary approach to managing insomnia and improving sleep quality. Here are some acupressure points for insomnia relief:

- **Spirit Gate (HT7):** Located on the palm side of the wrist, in the depression just below the pinky finger. Apply gentle pressure to this point to calm the mind and promote sleep.

- **Inner Gate (P6):** Found on the inner forearm, about two and a half finger-widths above the wrist crease. Massaging or applying pressure to this point can reduce anxiety and improve sleep.

- **Anmian (Extra Point):** This point is located behind the earlobe. Gently massage this area with your fingers to help relieve insomnia and promote relaxation.

- **Yintang (Extra Point):** Positioned between the eyebrows, slightly above the Third Eye Point (GV24.5). Apply gentle pressure to this point to calm the mind and reduce insomnia-related stress.

- **Heart 7 (HT7):** Located on the palm side of the wrist, in the depression just below the pinky finger. Massaging this point can help reduce anxiety and promote relaxation for better sleep.

6.5 Digestive Issues

Acupressure can aid in alleviating digestive issues, including indigestion, bloating, and nausea. Here are some acupressure points to address digestive discomfort:

- **Abdominal Sorrow (CV12):** Found on the midline of the abdomen, about four finger-widths above the navel. Gently apply pressure to this point to relieve indigestion and abdominal discomfort.

- **Three Mile Point (ST36):** Located about four finger-widths below the kneecap and one finger-width towards the

outside of the shinbone.
Stimulating this point can help
with digestion and reduce
bloating.

- **Sea of Energy (CV6):** As
  mentioned earlier, this point
  below the navel is beneficial for
  overall digestive health.
  Applying pressure to CV6 can
  improve digestion and reduce
  nausea.

- **Pericardium 6 (P6):** Found on
  the inner forearm, about two
  and a half finger-widths above
  the wrist crease. Massaging or
  applying pressure to this point
  can help relieve nausea and
  indigestion.

6.6 Common Cold and Allergies

Acupressure can provide relief from common cold symptoms and allergies by targeting points that support the immune system and alleviate congestion. Here are some acupressure points for these conditions:

- **Union Valley (LI4):** Situated in the webbing between the thumb and index finger on both hands. Stimulating this point can help with sinus congestion and cold symptoms.

- **Welcome Fragrance (LI20):** Located on both sides of the nose, at the base of the nostrils. Gently press these points to alleviate nasal congestion and improve breathing.

- **Heavenly Pillar (B10):** As mentioned earlier, this point on the back of the neck can help relieve congestion and promote respiratory health.

- **Inner Gate (P6):** Also mentioned earlier, this point on the inner forearm can help reduce nausea and improve overall comfort during illness.

It's important to note that while acupressure can provide relief for these conditions, it should not replace medical treatment when necessary. If you have severe or chronic symptoms, consult a healthcare professional for a comprehensive evaluation and treatment plan.

CHAPTER 7

Acupressure for Emotional Well-Being

Acupressure can be a valuable tool for promoting emotional well-being by helping to balance and regulate emotions. It can aid in reducing stress, anxiety, and emotional tension while fostering a sense of calm and relaxation.

7.1 Balancing Emotions

Emotional balance is essential for overall well-being, and acupressure can play a role in achieving and maintaining it. Here are some acupressure points and techniques to help balance emotions:

- **Heart 7 (HT7):** Located on the palm side of the wrist, in the depression just below the pinky finger. Massaging or applying pressure to this point can help calm the mind and reduce anxiety and stress.

- **Spirit Gate (HT7):** The Spirit Gate point is on the same location as Heart 7, making it effective for balancing emotions and promoting emotional stability.

- **Yintang (Extra Point):** Positioned between the eyebrows, slightly above the Third Eye Point (GV24.5). Applying gentle pressure to this point can help soothe the mind and alleviate emotional tension.

- **Third Eye Point (GV24.5):** As mentioned earlier, this point is located between the eyebrows and is effective for promoting mental clarity and emotional balance.

Balancing Emotions Using Acupressure:

1. **Find a Quiet Space:** Choose a peaceful environment where you can relax without distractions.

2. **Sit or Lie Down:** Get into a comfortable sitting or lying position. Ensure that your body is relaxed, and your posture is aligned.

3. **Deep Breathing:** Start with a few minutes of deep, slow breathing. Inhale deeply through your nose, allowing your abdomen to expand, and exhale slowly through your mouth. This will help calm your nervous system.

4. **Select an Acupoint:** Choose one of the acupoints mentioned above (Heart 7, Spirit Gate, Yintang, or Third Eye Point) based on your emotional needs.

5. **Apply Gentle Pressure:** Use your thumb or forefinger to apply gentle pressure to the selected acupoint. Begin with light pressure and gradually increase it as needed. The pressure should be firm enough to feel a slight discomfort or "good pain" but not painful.

6. **Circular Motion:** While maintaining pressure, use a small, clockwise circular motion over the acupoint. This circular motion helps activate the point and stimulate energy flow.

7. **Breathing and Visualization:** As you stimulate the acupoint, continue deep, slow breathing. Visualize any emotional tension or stress leaving your body with each exhale.

8. **Duration:** Hold the pressure on the acupoint for 1 to 3 minutes. During this time, focus on your breath and the sensation at the acupoint.

9. **Release Slowly:** After the recommended time, release the pressure slowly and gently.

Take a moment to rest and observe any changes in your emotional state.

10. **Repeat as Needed:** You can repeat this acupressure technique as needed to maintain emotional balance. You may also explore different acupoints to see which one works best for you.

Acupressure is a complementary practice and should not replace professional mental health treatment when needed. If you are experiencing severe or persistent emotional issues, consider consulting a qualified mental health professional for guidance and support.

7.2 Managing Stress and Depression

Acupressure can be a helpful component of stress and depression management, promoting relaxation and emotional well-being. Here are acupressure points and techniques for managing stress and depression:

- **Heart 7 (HT7):** Located on the palm side of the wrist, in the depression just below the pinky finger. Applying gentle pressure to this point can help reduce stress, anxiety, and depressive feelings.

- **Spirit Gate (HT7):** As mentioned earlier, the Spirit Gate point is effective for emotional balance and can assist in managing stress and depression.

- **Third Eye Point (GV24.5):**
Positioned between the eyebrows, this point can help clear the mind, reduce emotional tension, and alleviate symptoms of stress and depression.

- **Union Valley (LI4):** Situated in the webbing between the thumb and index finger on both hands. Massaging or applying pressure to this point can help relieve emotional stress and promote relaxation.

Managing Stress and Depression Using Acupressure:

1. **Prepare:** Find a quiet and comfortable space where you can relax. Sit or lie down in a comfortable position and take a few deep, calming breaths.

2. **Select an Acupoint:** Choose one of the acupoints mentioned above (Heart 7, Spirit Gate, Third Eye Point, or Union Valley) based on your emotional needs.

3. **Apply Gentle Pressure:** Use your thumb or forefinger to apply gentle pressure to the selected acupoint. Start with light pressure and gradually increase it if needed, ensuring it's comfortable but not painful.

4. **Circular Motion:** While maintaining pressure, use a small, clockwise circular motion over the acupoint. This motion helps activate the point and encourages emotional release.

5. **Deep Breathing:** Continue with deep, slow breathing throughout the acupressure practice. Inhale

deeply through your nose, and exhale slowly through your mouth.

6. **Visualize and Release:** As you stimulate the acupoint, visualize any stress or depressive feelings dissipating with each exhale. Focus on releasing tension and emotional burdens.

7. **Duration:** Hold the pressure and perform the circular motion for 1 to 3 minutes, maintaining a relaxed state.

8. **Release Slowly:** After the recommended time, release the pressure slowly and gently. Take a moment to rest and observe any changes in your emotional state.

9. **Repeat as Needed:** You can repeat this acupressure technique whenever you feel stressed, anxious, or depressed. Experiment

with different acupoints to determine which one provides the most relief for you.

7.3 Building Self-awareness

Acupressure can also be a tool for building self-awareness and promoting emotional insight. While acupressure points can help alleviate emotional tension, the practice itself can encourage mindfulness and self-reflection. Here's how to use acupressure for building self-awareness:

1. **Select an Acupoint:** Choose an acupoint based on your emotional state and the specific area you want to focus on. Consider points

like Third Eye Point (GV24.5), Spirit Gate (HT7), or Yintang.

2. **Apply Gentle Pressure:** As previously described, apply gentle pressure to the selected acupoint with your thumb or forefinger. Start with light pressure and gradually increase it as needed.

3. **Mindful Sensation:** As you stimulate the acupoint, pay close attention to the physical sensations and feelings that arise. Notice any warmth, tingling, or relaxation in the area.

4. **Breath Awareness:** Concentrate on your breath during the acupressure practice. Observe the rhythm of your breath and how it may change as you apply pressure to the point.

5. **Emotional Reflection:** While practicing acupressure, allow your mind to wander and explore your emotions. Use this time for self-reflection and self-awareness. Consider any thoughts or feelings that come to the surface.

6. **Journaling:** After the acupressure session, consider journaling your thoughts and emotions. Write down any insights or revelations that occurred during the practice. This can help you gain a deeper understanding of your emotional patterns.

7. **Consistency:** Make acupressure for self-awareness a regular practice. Over time, it can help you develop greater emotional intelligence and insight into your own well-being.

Acupressure can be a valuable tool for promoting self-awareness, understanding emotional triggers, and managing stress and depression. When used in combination with mindfulness and self-reflection, it can contribute to improved emotional well-being and overall mental health.

CHAPTER 8

Incorporating Acupressure into Daily Life

Acupressure can be a beneficial practice when integrated into your daily routine, promoting overall well-being and balance.

8.1 Creating a Routine

Establishing a daily acupressure routine can help you reap the full benefits of this practice. Here's a step-by-step guide to creating a routine:

Step 1: Set Goals

Determine your goals for incorporating acupressure into your daily life. Are you seeking stress relief, pain management, emotional balance, or general wellness? Knowing your objectives will guide your practice.

Step 2: Identify Key Acupoints

Research and identify acupoints that align with your goals. Make a list of these points and their locations. You can reference acupressure charts, books, or consult a qualified acupressure practitioner for guidance.

Step 3: Allocate Time

Decide how much time you can dedicate to acupressure each day. Even just a few minutes can be beneficial. Choose a specific time, such as morning or evening, to incorporate acupressure into your routine.

Step 4: Start Small

Begin with a manageable number of acupoints. You don't need to work on all of them at once. Start with a few key points that align with your goals and gradually expand your routine as you become more comfortable.

Step 5: Create a Relaxing Environment

Select a quiet and peaceful space where you can practice acupressure without distractions. Dim the lights, play calming music, or diffuse essential oils to enhance the relaxation experience.

Step 6: Practice Mindfulness

Before starting your acupressure routine, take a moment to center yourself. Practice mindfulness and deep breathing to prepare your mind and body for the session.

Step 7: Perform Acupressure

Follow the techniques described in earlier sections to apply pressure to the selected acupoints. Use circular motions, rhythmic pressure, and deep breathing to enhance the effectiveness of your practice.

Step 8: Observe Changes

After your acupressure session, take a moment to notice any changes in your physical or emotional state. This self-awareness can help you gauge the effectiveness of your routine.

Step 9: Adjust and Expand

Based on your observations and goals, adjust your routine as needed. You can gradually add more acupoints, increase the duration, or explore different techniques to enhance your practice.

Step 10: Be Consistent

Consistency is key to experiencing the long-term benefits of acupressure. Commit to your daily routine and make it a habit in your daily life.

8.2 Self-Care Tips

Incorporating acupressure into your daily life is a form of self-care that can promote physical and emotional well-being. Here are additional self-care tips to complement your acupressure practice:

1. **Healthy Lifestyle:** Maintain a balanced diet, engage in regular physical activity, stay hydrated, and prioritize adequate sleep. A

healthy lifestyle supports the effectiveness of acupressure.

2. **Mindfulness Meditation:** Combine acupressure with mindfulness meditation to enhance relaxation and self-awareness. Meditation can complement your acupressure practice and promote emotional balance.

3. **Hydrotherapy:** Consider warm baths, hot or cold compresses, or contrast showers as complementary treatments to enhance the effects of acupressure.

4. **Stretching Exercises:** Incorporate gentle stretching exercises into your daily routine to improve flexibility, reduce muscle tension, and enhance the benefits of acupressure.

5. **Stress Management:** Implement stress management techniques such as deep breathing, progressive muscle relaxation, and guided imagery alongside acupressure for greater stress relief.

6. **Journaling:** Keep a journal to track your acupressure sessions, emotional changes, and insights gained from the practice. This can help you fine-tune your routine and monitor your progress.

7. **Consult a Professional:** If you have specific health concerns or conditions, consider consulting a qualified acupressure practitioner or healthcare provider for personalized guidance and treatment.

8. **Self-Compassion:** Practice self-compassion and kindness toward yourself. Understand that self-care, including acupressure, is a form of self-love and nurturing.

Incorporating acupressure into your daily life, along with these self-care tips, can contribute to improved physical and emotional well-being. Remember that acupressure is a holistic approach to wellness and complements other healthy habits and practices.

8.3 Combining Acupressure with Other Practices

Combining acupressure with other complementary practices can enhance its effectiveness and contribute to a holistic approach to health and well-being. Here are several practices you can combine with acupressure for a well-rounded approach to self-care:

1. Yoga: Yoga combines physical postures, breathing exercises, and meditation to promote flexibility, relaxation, and mental clarity. Combining acupressure with yoga can help address both physical and emotional concerns, such as muscle tension and stress.

2. Meditation and Mindfulness: Meditation and mindfulness practices promote relaxation, self-awareness, and stress reduction. Incorporating mindfulness techniques with acupressure can enhance the overall calming effect and emotional balance.

3. Aromatherapy: Essential oils from aromatherapy can complement acupressure by providing pleasant scents and promoting relaxation. Use diffusers or diluted essential oils during your acupressure sessions to create a soothing atmosphere.

4. Herbal Remedies: Herbal remedies and supplements can be used alongside acupressure to address specific health concerns. Consult with a qualified herbalist or healthcare provider to ensure safety and effectiveness.

5. Tai Chi: Tai Chi is a gentle and flowing form of exercise that promotes balance, flexibility, and relaxation. It can be integrated with acupressure to enhance overall well-being and promote the free flow of energy (Qi) in the body.

6. Physical Therapy: If you have specific physical conditions or injuries, working with a physical therapist in conjunction with acupressure can provide comprehensive care for rehabilitation and pain management.

7. Nutritional Support: A balanced diet plays a crucial role in overall health. Combining acupressure with proper nutrition can support your body's healing processes and energy balance.

8. Breathing Exercises: Deep breathing exercises, such as pranayama in yoga, can be integrated with acupressure to enhance relaxation and oxygenate the body for better healing.

9. Reflexology: Reflexology is a practice that focuses on specific points on the feet and hands. Combining acupressure with reflexology can provide a comprehensive approach to promoting well-being and relaxation.

10. Guided Imagery: Incorporating guided imagery or visualization techniques during acupressure sessions can help you set intentions and enhance the healing process.

11. Traditional Chinese Medicine (TCM): Consider consulting a TCM practitioner who can provide dietary recommendations, herbal remedies, and acupuncture treatments alongside acupressure for a holistic approach to health.

12. Chiropractic Care: Chiropractic adjustments and acupressure can work together to address musculoskeletal issues and promote overall physical comfort.

13. Energy Healing: Practices like Reiki, qigong, or energy healing modalities can be combined with acupressure to balance and harmonize the body's energy systems.

When combining acupressure with other practices, it's essential to ensure that they complement each other and align with your specific health goals and needs. Consult with qualified practitioners or healthcare providers as needed to create a personalized and effective holistic wellness plan.